Alkaline Foods-100% Raw Easy and Tasty Raw Food Recipes Including Alkaline Salads, Smoothies and Treats!

By Marta Tuchowska

Copyright ©Marta Tuchowska

2015, 2016

www.HolisticWellnessProject.com

"HOW TO INCORPORATE MORE ALKALINE RAW FOODS INTO YOUR DIET TO ENJOY HIGH ENERGY LEVELS, HOLISTIC WELLNESS, AND NATURAL WEIGHT LOSS.

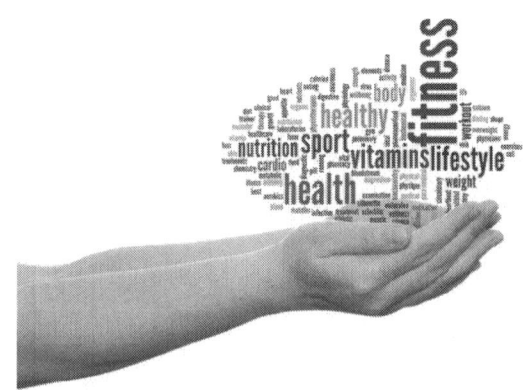

All rights reserved. No part of this publication may be reproduced, stored in a retrieval system, or transmitted, in any form or by any means, electronic, mechanical, photocopying, recording or otherwise, without the prior written permission of the author and the publishers.

The scanning, uploading, and distribution of this book via the Internet, or via any other means, without the permission of the author is illegal and punishable by law. Please purchase only authorized electronic editions, and do not participate in or encourage electronic piracy of copyrighted materials.

All information in this book has been carefully researched and checked for factual accuracy. However, the author and publishers make no warranty, expressed or implied, that the information contained herein is appropriate for every individual, situation or purpose, and assume no responsibility for errors or omission. The reader assumes the risk and full responsibility for all actions, and the author will not be held liable for any loss or damage, whether consequential, incidental, and special or otherwise, that may result from the information presented in this publication.

A physician has not written the information in this book. Before making any serious dietary changes, I advise you to consult with your physician first.

Contents

From the Author 7
More Benefits of Raw Foods 11
The Alkaline Diet- The Common Sense Approach....12
Alkaline Diet Crash Course- Understand the Basics 20
Disclaimer 23
RECIPES 24
   Natural Detox Carrot Soup 24
   Natural Protein Smoothie 26
   Energy Lover Smoothie 28
   Kale Smoothie for Skeptics 30
   Spicy Exotic Smoothie Soup Style 33
   Sprout-y Salad with an Exotic Twist 35
   Raw Veggie Noodles 38
   Coconut Gazpacho-Style Raw Veggie Cream 40
   Almost Raw Curry 42
   Alkaline Raw Green Energy Juice 44
   Liver Lover Green-ish Juice 46
   Refreshing Mango Blend 48
   Delicious Choco-Vegan Shake 50
   Body and Mind Energizing Roibos Berry Treat 51
   Sweet Choco-Avo Pudding 53
   Raw Orange Ice-Cream 54
   Vegan Raw Brownies 55
   Amazing Alkaline Ginger Cookies 57

Raw Coconut Milk 61
Raw Carrot Cookies 63
Apple and Celery Root Salad 65
Summer Veggies Party 67
Green Papaya Salad Spiced Up 69
Rainbow Raw Salad 71
Papaya Guacamole Spiced Up 74
Healthy Eyes Raw Juice 76
Drink It Up- Health Shot! 78
Holiday Feeling Tropical Anti-Inflammatory Juice 82
Longevity Sweet Juice 2 in 1 Recipe 85
BONUS Recipe- What to do with a pulp? 86
Mango Mustard Salad 88
More Delicious Salad Dressings and Salsas 90
CONCLUSION 92

From the Author

Dear Reader! Thank you so much for taking an interest in my book. My goal is to provide you with simple and effective natural tools for wellness and natural weight loss including solutions that you can apply even if you are on a busy schedule, like myself. If you want more energy and vibrant health, you have come to the right place. Forget about the latest fad diets and simply focus on enriching your existing diet with real foods. Your body and mind will be utterly grateful! I am very excited to show you how to do just that- create amazing, mouth-watering dishes that are relatively quick and easy to prepare. I also want to stimulate your imagination and creativity so that you can start inventing your own recipes.

Raw food lifestyle is very flexible and open-minded. It means that it doesn't matter if you are vegan, vegetarian, paleo, alkaline, gluten-free, or you don't follow anything at all. You can always add more raw foods into your diet!

Read on with an open mind and make sure you practice what you have learned. The recipes from this book are really easy and quick to make. You do not need to spend hundreds of dollars, euros, pounds (or whatever currency you use in your country) on expensive superfood fads. The solution is just in front of you.

In case you have not read my book "Raw Food Diet," the following paragraphs will quickly sum up and explain all the benefits to eating a raw food diet.

I also have a free, complimentary eBook that I have created to help you in your health and wellness journey. It's one of my most popular healthy recipe books so far, and I am giving it to you for free. Aside from the actual recipes, you will learn a few simple rules of alkaline and acidic foods as well as pH balancing. Again, it doesn't matter what dietary lifestyle you already follow. An alkaline diet lifestyle is very similar to a raw foods lifestyle, and everyone can benefit by transitioning their diet to a more natural, wholesome way. Find out more by grabbing your free copy (2 Bonus eBooks) today. Check them out at:

www.holisticwellnessproject.com/alkaline

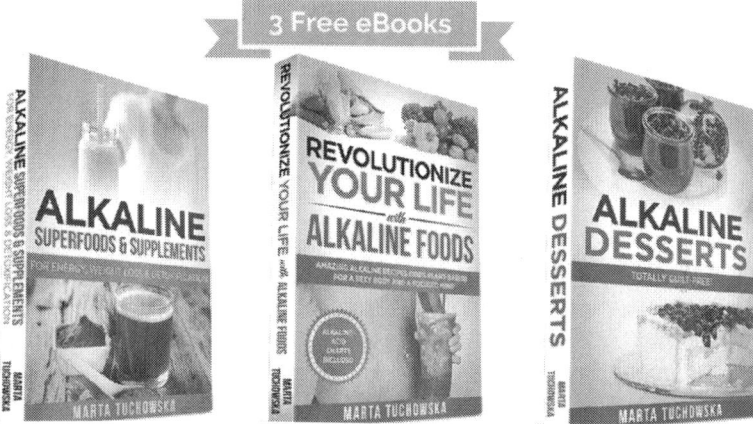

Now, back to raw foods!

The basic rundown of this simple diet is:

- The raw food diet, as the name suggests, promotes eating foods that are unprocessed and uncooked, such as fruits, vegetables, nuts, seeds, herbs.
- Some raw foodists, who are not vegan or vegetarian, also include some raw fish, eggs, as well as raw milk and fermented foods (unpasteurized) like for example, kefir or kombucha. Personally, when it comes to eating raw, I like the vegan approach as much as possible (and my recipes are focused on vegan raw foods).

- Raw foods are not necessarily 100% raw, some raw foodists cook their foods, but the basic rule is that the temperatures should not be higher than 40 degrees Celsius (or: 104 degrees Farenheit). Most of my recipes are 100% raw, but in some cases, I go through the slight cooking process.

6 simple reasons why raw foods are good for you:

- Excessive cooking kills the nutrients as well as many enzymes (these are responsible for proper digestion), and so if there are no raw foods in your diet, you are more likely to experience low energy levels and fatigue as well as sluggish digestion (after a cooked meal you usually feel sleepy, right?).
- Raw fruits and vegetables are an excellent sources of natural dietary fiber, hence the natural weight loss benefit.
- Raw foods will nourish your body with tons of vitamins and minerals that are crucial for beautiful skin and hair
- You will improve your digestion
- You will stimulate natural healing
- You will stimulate your immune system

More Benefits of Raw Foods

- easy to prepare
- excellent source of energy for the summer
- can be combined with any other diet that you have chosen to follow
- provide you with endless possibilities as for tasty and sweet desserts, and can help you control food cravings.

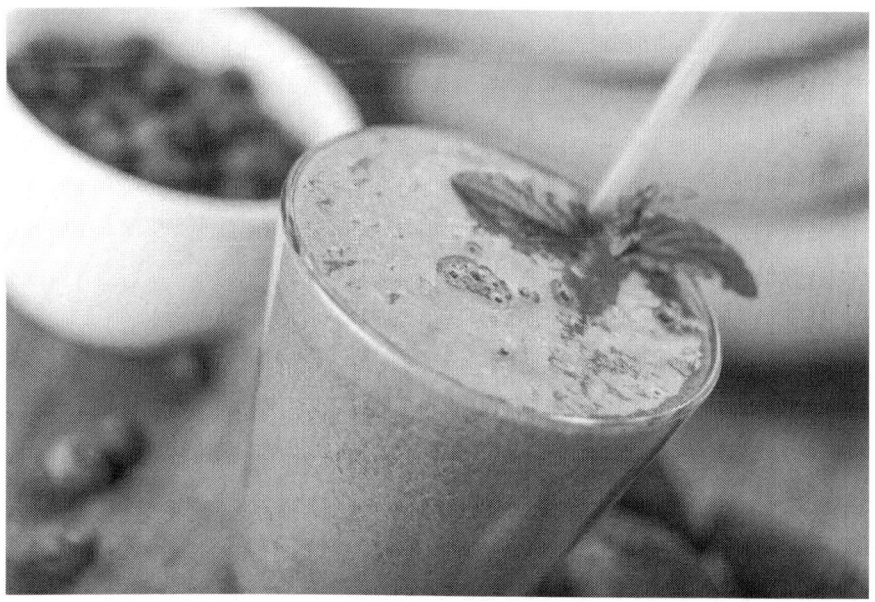

This is a practical recipe book for modern people who would like to experiment a little bit with "raw-fooding" and increase their energy levels and quality of life. You don't have to go vegan or raw-food 100% (unless you want to, then I will give you all my support), just like I am not telling you to follow a given diet. I am trying to encourage you to create your own healthy nutrition habits. The raw food diet is one of the tools that I would like to explain in this book. Your homework will be to find your own way and see what works for you.

Now...let's get the basics of the alkaline diet...

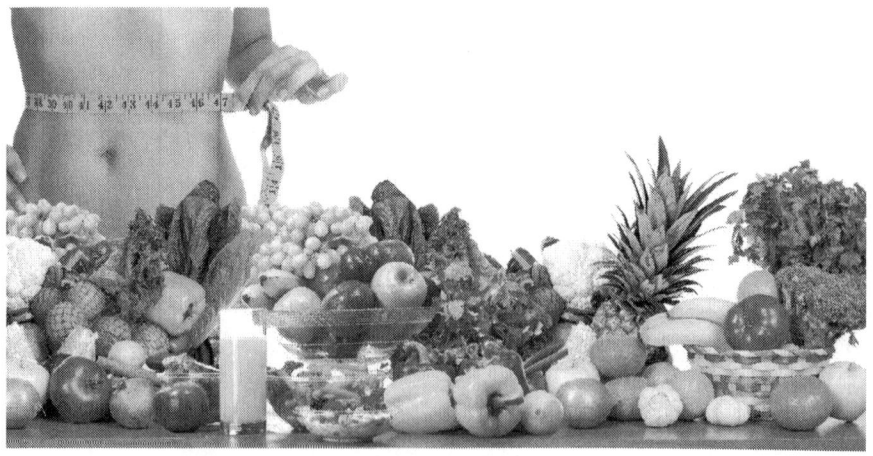

The Alkaline Diet- The Common Sense Approach

The alkaline diet is a lifestyle that encourages you to give your body the nourishment it needs so that it can work for you at its optimal levels without feeling too exhausted or too acidic. Too much acidity in the body is leading to depression, sickness, and obesity.

Dr. Robert O' Young, Director of Research at the pH Miracle Living Center, says that your fat may be protecting your very life against the acidity in your body. He goes on to make this bold statement.

"There is only one disease: The Constant Acidification of the Body."

What this means is that every disease, including excess weight, is because of a body that is too acidic. These things can make your body too acidic: processed foods, sugar, foods containing gluten and yeast, meat and animal products, stress, alcohol, tobacco, drugs, caffeine, and pollution.

Luckily, the alkaline diet gives us natural tools to fix the problem. I am not talking about overpriced superfoods from overseas that are difficult to find and to pronounce. The simplest methods are always the best and you will be surprised by how healthy you will feel by adding more everyday healing, alkaline foods into your diet (even if you don't follow a strict alkaline diet).

If you attend the root cause of the problem, by implementing a lifestyle rich in alkaline forming foods, it will naturally take care of what plagues you.

Here are a few simple guidelines that will help you transition towards a healthy, alkaline lifestyle. These are compatible with different nutritional lifestyles (Gluten Free, Vegetarian, Vegan) and it's totally up to you what you choose to focus on:

1) **Eliminate processed foods from your diet and say "no" to colas and sodas** - there are so many additives and preservatives in these foods. They have been known to create hormone imbalances, make you tired, and add to acidity in your body. It's just not natural for humans to consume those conveniently processed foods. The label may even say "low in calories or low in fat"- it will not help you in your long term weight loss or health efforts. In order to start losing weight naturally, your body needs foods that are jam-

packed with nutrients. Real foods. Living foods. This, in turn, will help your body maintain its optimal blood pH (7.35) almost effortlessly.

2) **Add more raw foods into your diet**- THIS IS WHAT THIS BOOK IS ALL ABOUT- especially lots of vegetables and leafy greens as well as fruits that are naturally low in sugar (for example, limes, lemons, grapefruits, avocados, tomatoes, and pomegranates are alkaline forming fruits).

3) **Reduce/eliminate animal products** – these are extremely acid-forming. The good news is that there are many plant-based options out there and tons of way to create delicious alkaline-friendly plant-based meals you will love! If I could do it, you can do it too.

4) **Drink plenty of clean, filtered water**, preferably alkaline water or fruit-infused water.

5) **Add more vegetable juices into your diet**- these are a great way to give your body more nutrients and alkalinity that will result in more energy, less inflammation and, if desired- natural weight loss. Vegetable juices are the best shots of health! I have

written a bestselling book on alkaline juicing if want to give it a try and want to juice the right way.

6) **Reduce/eliminate processed grains, "crappy carbs" as well as yeast** (very acid-forming). Personally, I recommend quinoa instead (it's naturally gluten-free), amaranth (very nutritious), brown rice, or soba noodles (it's made from buckwheat and naturally gluten-free). You can also use gluten-free wraps or make your own bread. Fruit is also a great natural source of carbohydrates, and great for energy. Plus, they always make a great snack!

7) **Reduce/eliminate caffeine**- trust me - it will only make you feel sick and tired in the long run, and can even lead to adrenal exhaustion (not the best condition to end up in - I have been there). It may seem a bit drastic at first, and yes, I know what you're thinking- there are so many articles out there praising benefits of caffeine and coffee. Yes, I am sure there are, as many people build their business around coffee. This is why there must be something out there that promotes it. At the same time, I agree that everything is good for you in moderation. As long as you have a healthy foundation, you can have coffee as a treat (I do drink coffee occasionally). There is no reason to be too strict on

yourself. But...don't rely on caffeine as your main source of energy. Green tea may be helpful too as a transition, but green tea is not caffeine-free either so don't overdo it. On the other side of spectrum - green tea is rich in antioxidants and a great part of a balanced diet, so it's not that you have to get paranoid about all kinds of caffeine. <u>Moderation is the key</u>. Try to observe your body. Personally, I have noticed that quitting my coffee habits (I used to have 2-3 coffees a day) and replacing coffee with natural herbal teas and infusions have really made my energy levels skyrocket. Now I sleep better, and I get up feeling nice and fresh. I don't need caffeine to keep me awake. I no longer suffer from tension headaches and I feel calmer. Yes, I do have a cup of coffee as a treat sometimes, usually when I meet with a friend, but I no longer depend on it. I choose it; it doesn't choose me. Think about this and how you can apply this simple tip to your life to achieve total wellbeing. Coffee and caffeine in general is extremely acid-forming.

I recently started using an Ayurvedic herb called Ashwagandha. It is known as an adaptogenic herb and it can help you restore your energy levels naturally. I highly recommend you give it a try!

8) **Replace cow's milk with almond milk, coconut milk or any other vegan friendly milk** (for example quinoa milk, chia seed milk, oats milk- whatever works for you and your stomach) that works well for you. Cow's milk is extremely acid forming and personally, I don't think it makes sense for humans to drink milk that is naturally designed for fattening baby calves not humans. Actually, quitting dairy was one of the best things I have done for myself. I have noticed that even very little milk would cause digestive problems and it was really easy to fix-I quit drinking milk. I also learned about cruelty in the dairy industry which obviously contributed to my decision. The best thing about the alkaline plant-based diet is that you can still have ice cream and other treats- you just make them with no milk/animal products. It's so much healthier and tastier, totally guilt-free. With this approach, there is no need to go hungry or deprived. You focus on abundance of foods and meals that are good for you, delicious and such a choice is also better for the animals and the planet. This is what I call- holistic motivation.

9) **Don't fear good fats- coconut oil, olive oil, avocado oil** etc. are good for you and should replace processed margarines, and artery-clogging trans-fats.

This is not to say that you can "drink" them freely. Balance is the key.

Also...

Use stevia instead of processed sugar (stevia is sweet but sugar-free) and Himalayan salt instead of regular salt (Himalayan salt contain some amounts of calcium, iron, potassium and magnesium plus it also contains lower amounts of sodium than regular salt.)

Add more spices and herbs into your diet- not only do they make your dishes taste amazing but they also have anti-inflammatory properties and help you detoxify (cilantro, turmeric, and cinnamon are miraculous).

As you can see, the alkaline diet is a pretty common sense clean diet. Nothing is exaggerated. Nothing is too strict. Nothing is too faddish. Eat more living foods and avoid processed foods. Try to eat more plant based foods. Don't reject it before you have tried it.

Alkaline Diet Crash Course- Understand the Basics

The pH of most of our important cellular and other fluids (like blood) is actually designed to be at pH of 7.35 (slightly alkaline).

The body has an intricate system in place to always maintain that healthy, slightly alkaline pH level – no matter what you eat. This is an argument that many alkaline diet skeptics use and I get it. It's 100% true.

This is not the goal of the alkaline diet. We just can't make our blood's pH more alkaline or "higher." Our body tries to work really hard for us to help us maintain our ideal pH (7.35). We can't have a pH of 8 or 9. If we did we would be dead.

The entire focus of the alkaline diet is to give your body the nourishment and healing tools it needs to MAINTAIN that optimal 7.35 pH almost effortlessly.

If we fail to do so, we torture our body with an incredible stress! Yes- when the body has to constantly work overtime to detoxify all the cells and maintain our pH it finally succumbs to disease.

Let me just name a few cases of what can happen if we constantly eat an acid-forming diet (also called SAD - Standard American Diet) that is not supporting our body at all. Our body ends up sick and tired of working overtime and may manifest one or more of the following conditions:

-constant inflammation

-immune and hormone imbalance

-lack of energy, mental fog

-yeast and candida overgrowth

 -digestive damage

-weakened bones (our body is forced to pull minerals like magnesium and calcium from our bones in order to maintain alkaline balance it needs for constant healing processes).

In summary, eating more alkaline foods helps support our body so that it can work for us at optimal levels while eating more acidic food doesn't help at all. The alkaline diet is not about magically raising our pH but helping our body rebalance itself by supporting its natural healing functions.

I hope you're feeling excited about re-energizing your body and mind with the most nutritious, raw, alkaline foods.

Let's get right into it...

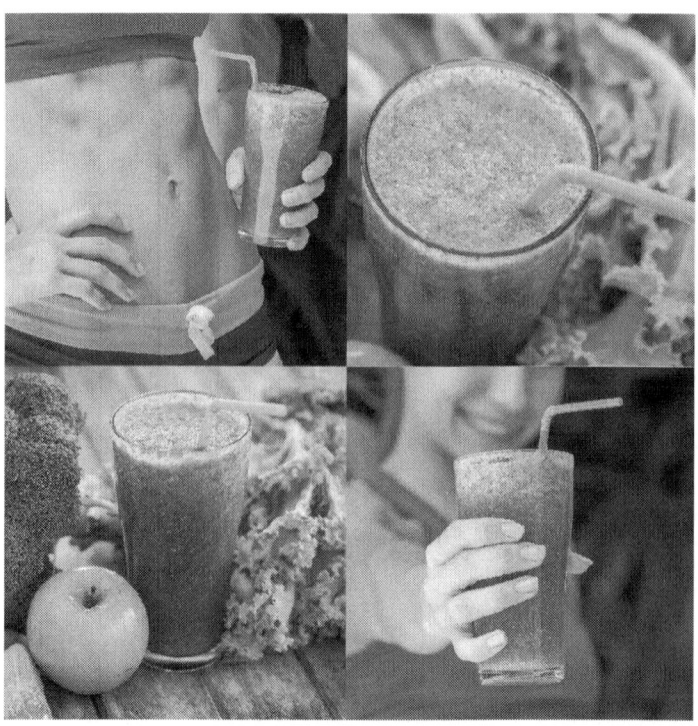

Disclaimer

All cooking is an experiment in a sense, and many people come to the same or similar recipe over time. All recipes in this book have been derived from author's personal experience. Should any bear a close resemblance to those used elsewhere, that is purely coincidental.

The book is not intended to provide medical advice or to take the place of medical advice and treatment from your personal physician. Readers are advised to consult their own doctors or other qualified health professionals regarding the treatment of medical conditions. The author shall not be held liable or responsible for any misunderstanding or misuse of the information contained in this book. The information is not intended to diagnose, treat or cure any disease.

It is important to remember that the author of this book is not a doctor/ medical professional. Only opinions based upon her own personal experiences or research are cited. THE AUTHOR DOES NOT OFFER MEDICAL ADVICE or prescribe any treatments. For any health or medical issues – you should be talking to your doctor first.

RECIPES

Natural Detox Carrot Soup

This recipe will help boost your immune system with massive amounts of vitamins C and A. Ginger is great for digestive problems and acts as a natural anti-inflammatory. You can experiment to make this soup a bit denser so that it's more like a cream or a dip. It's up to you.

Serves: 2

Ingredients:

- 4 large carrots (peeled unless organic) and chopped
- Juice of 1 orange
- 1 mango, peeled, pitted and chopped
- 2 inches of ginger
- 1 big onion
- 1 red bell pepper
- 2 garlic cloves
- ½ cup cilantro, chopped
- 2 cups coconut milk
- 1 tablespoon olive oil
- ¼ cup sunflower seeds
- Himalayan salt to taste

Instructions:

1. Place all the ingredients (except cilantro, sunflower seeds and oil) in a blender. Blend until smooth and creamy.
2. Add a pinch of Himalayan salt to taste. Sprinkle some olive oil, cilantro and sunflower seeds over the soup.
3. Enjoy!

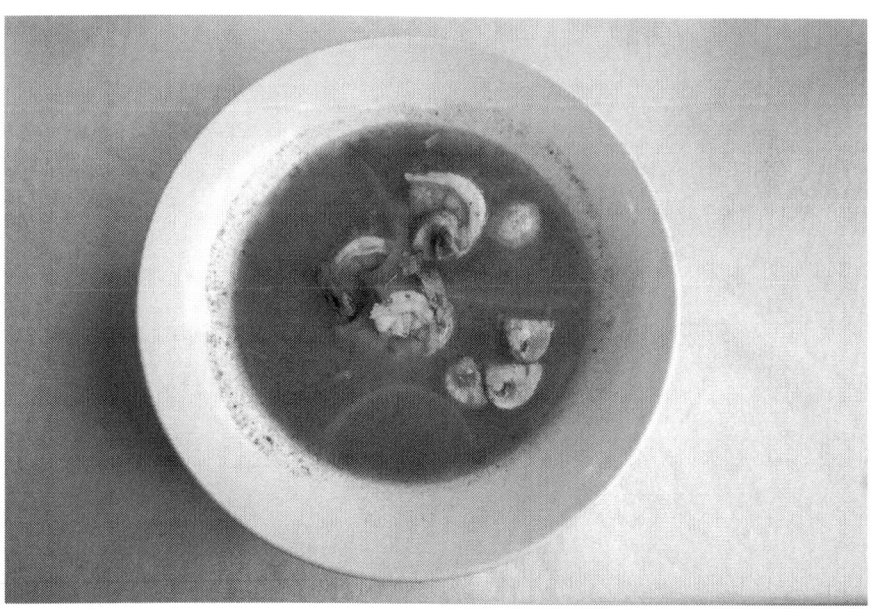

Natural Protein Smoothie

I really recommend this smoothie to all fitness enthusiasts and body builders who are inspired by the vegan and vegetarian lifestyle. Even if you are not planning to become a full-time vegan, you can always do it part-time and give your body a break from animal products. Green leafy veggies, nuts and seeds are just perfect! Lemon or grapefruit juice will help alkalize your body even further which will result in higher energy levels. You want to feel light and energized, not heavy, right? There is no need to resort to artificial energy or sports drinks that only mess with your hormones and fill you with toxins...

Serves: 2

Ingredients:

- 2 cups of raw organic almond milk
- 1 cup filtered water
- 2 bananas
- 1 tablespoon of chia seeds
- 1 cup of soy sprouts
- ¼ cup peanuts
- ½ cup kale leaves
- Juice of 2 lemons (or 1 grapefruit)
- 1 teaspoon of ginger powder

- 1 tablespoon of coconut oil

Instructions:

Place in a blender, blend well, and enjoy!

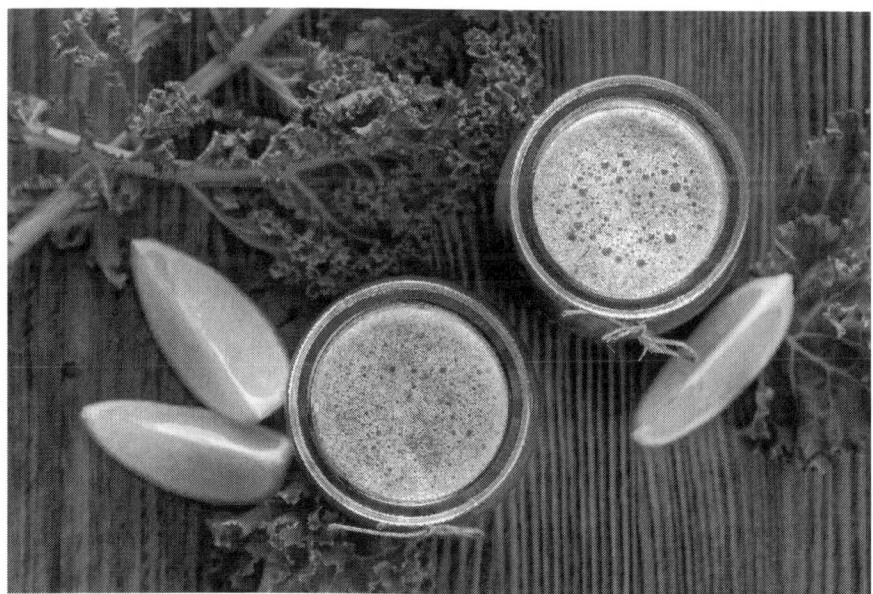

Energy Lover Smoothie

Energize your body and mind with this nutrient-dense, delicious tasting smoothie. Don't forget about the secret ingredient- the maca powder. So what is it? Well, according to the legend, it's an aphrodisiac. It's enough to look at maca's impressive nutritional value (great source of Vitamin B6, Potassium, Manganese, Vitamin C, Iron and Copper) to come to a simple conclusion- spice up your smoothies, juices, and even soups with some maca powder!

Ginger is a natural anti-inflammatory. It also has pH balancing properties (so have avocado, coconut water, almonds and mint leaves). Banana is a natural source of energy (don't worry about calories), and blueberries are a fantastic antioxidant. Drink your way to health!

Serves: 2

Ingredients:

- A few mint leaves
- 2 bananas
- 1 avocado
- ½ cup blueberries

- ¼ cup almonds (soaked in water for at least 8 hours)
- 2 cups of coconut water
- 1 tsp. maca powder
- ½ teaspoon ginger powder

Instructions:

Place in a blender and blend until smooth. Enjoy!

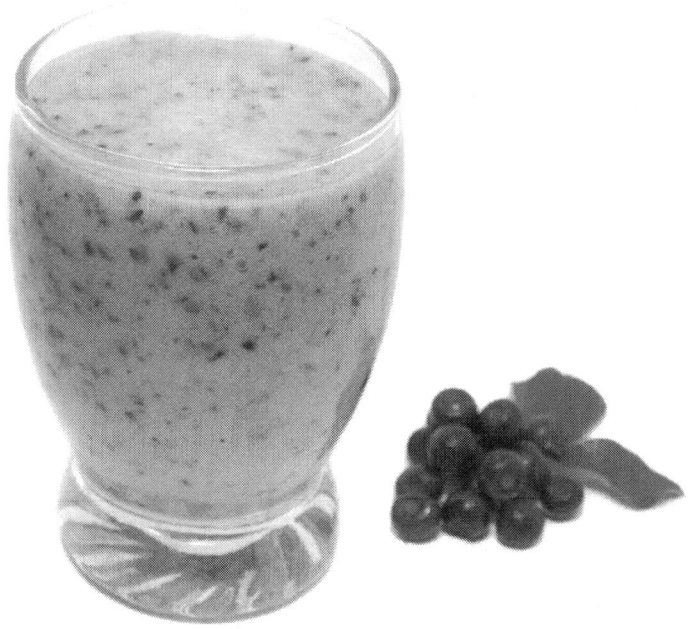

Kale Smoothie for Skeptics

You have probably heard that adding more greens into your diet will do wonders to your overall health and energy levels. All green, chlorophyll rich foods, especially leafy veggies, are good for you. However, very few people feel naturally attracted to them. This is why it's a good idea to mix them with some other ingredients. Your green smoothie will taste delicious, so that it's not torture for you to go more green and alkaline. Success with foods and diets is pretty much like success in your professional life; it's always better to do something you at least slightly enjoy, right?

Coconut milk is an excellent vegan milk option. It's low in cholesterol, low in sodium, and rich in Manganese (this mineral takes care of your sex hormones, brain, fat and carbohydrate metabolism, calcium absorption, and bones). It also has alkalizing benefits. I often hear people worry about calories. Forget about this old-fashioned concept. Focus on nutrients, real foods, and more raw foods (this is what you are already doing because you have picked up this book). Even if you are not a vegan, try to learn more vegan options. To wrap up- you will be better drinking good quality organic, unsweetened coconut milk or almond milk rather than super acidic cow's milk, which is probably packed with hormones, even though it's labeled as "low fat". Fats that come from natural foods like coconut oil and other coconut products (avocados, nuts, seeds, olive oil, etc.) are good for you. So don't fear them, and don't fear real foods, even if they have a few more calories. Besides, counting calories only takes away your emotional wellness. Been there, done that, not for me. Of course, I am not telling you what to do; the final choice is yours. But, I wish someone had told me this stuff when I was in my early twenties when I was obsessed about low fat and low calories and knew very little about the real secret to genuine health and natural weight loss. The secret is to eat real foods. Look what nature has to offer!

Serves: 2

Ingredients:

- 2 cups of raw, organic, unsweetened coconut milk
- 2 peaches (or pears)
- 1 green apple
- 1 cup of kale leaves
- pinch of cinnamon
- pinch of nutmeg
- 1/4 cup of dried fruits of your choice (for example raisins)

Instructions:

Place in a blender and enjoy!

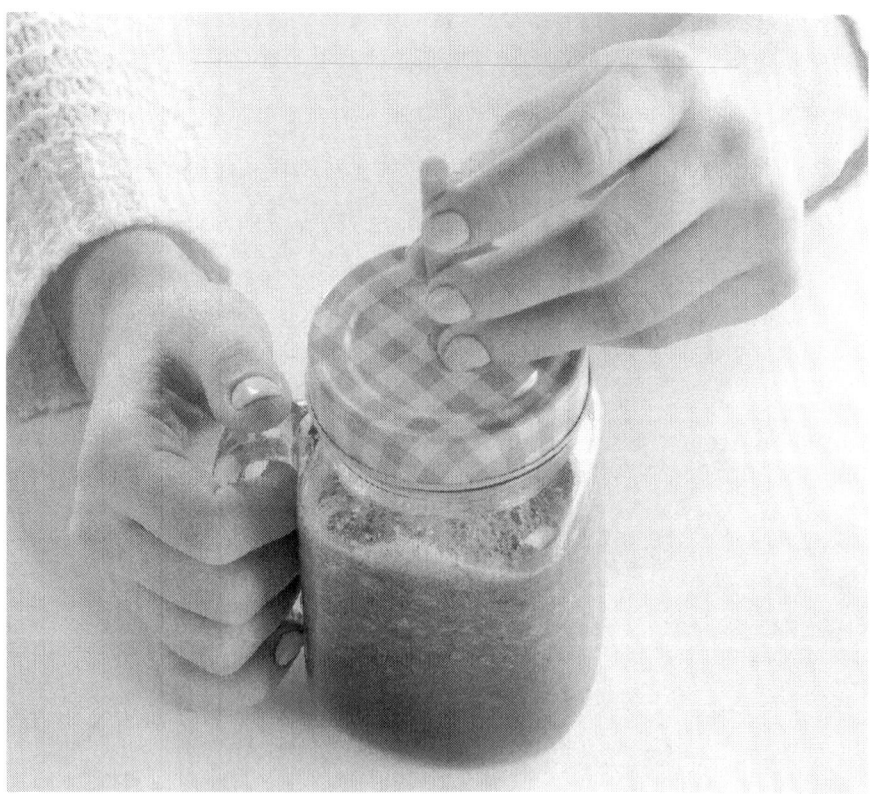

Spicy Exotic Smoothie Soup Style

I love cilantro! It gives an amazing, exotic flavor to all my dishes including smoothies. However, it's not only about the taste. I also like the fact that it acts as a natural antioxidant and aids in body detoxification (making you feel nice and fresh!). To sum up- it's a great herb, and curries are not the only way to take advantage of it. Now when it comes to smoothies, most people would naturally think of fruits. Don't get me wrong. I am all for fruit, but there is so much more to explore. Vegetables and greens are super alkalizing so use them in your smoothies. You can use your blender to create nutrient-packed, dense smoothies almost like soups or vegetable creams. They are quick and easy to prepare and a fantastic way of eating in the summer. In the winter, you may heat them up slightly, but remember that if you want to keep it in raw-foodish way, you should not exceed 100° Fahrenheit.

Serves: 2

Ingredients:

- 1 cup coconut milk
- 2 cups filtered water (preferably alkaline water)
- 1/4 cup cilantro
- 1/2 cup spinach leaves

- 1 zucchini
- 2 garlic cloves
- ½ cup of radish
- 1/4 cup of cashews (soaked in water for a few hours)
- 1/2 tsp. turmeric powder
- 1/4 tsp black pepper (real game changer as it helps your body get all the anti-inflammatory benefits that turmeric powder offers)
- 1/4 Himalayan salt
- 1 tablespoon organic, cold-pressed, virgin olive oil

Instructions:

1. Blend well, squeeze some fresh lime or lemon juice into the mixture, and enjoy!
2. Serve cold or slightly heated (but keep it raw).

Sprout-y Salad with an Exotic Twist

Want to have healthy skin, nails, and hair? Add more alfalfa sprouts and other sprouts into your diet. Just look at the nutritional value that speaks for itself:

-raw alfalfa sprouts are rich in Protein, Vitamin A, Calcium, Niacin, Vitamin C, Vitamin K, Thiamin, Riboflavin, Folate, Pantothenic Acid, Iron, Magnesium, Phosphorus, Zinc, Copper and Manganese

-soybean sprouts will revitalize your body and mind with natural Protein, Thiamin, Magnesium, Phosphorus, Copper, Potassium, Vitamin C, Folate and Manganese.

You can also use alfalfa powder supplements; they blend well with smoothies and juices.

Now the question is, how do you make sprouts appealing, tasty, and fun to eat? It's simple- follow my recipe! You can prepare this delicious, exotic salsa and store it in your fridge. Whenever you feel like snacking, just take some salsa and spread over the sprouts and nuts. It will only take a few seconds. So no excuses- healthy eating is easy. This is the healthiest and the rawest version of fast food!

Serves: 2

Ingredients (Salad):

- 1 cup of soybean sprouts
- 1 cup of alfalfa sprouts
- 1 cucumber
- ½ cup of almonds
- 1 apple, sliced
- ¼ onion, sliced

Ingredients (Salsa):

- ¼ cup coconut milk
- 2 tablespoons of olive oil
- Juice of 1 lemon
- 1 garlic clove, minced
- A few cilantro leaves
- Pinch of Himalayan salt
- Pinch of black pepper
- Pinch of curry powder

Instructions:

1. Mix all the salsa ingredients in a small bowl or a cup.

2. Prepare the salad in a bowl and spread the salsa over the delicious spicy salad.
3. Enjoy! It's really healthy, refreshing, mineralizing and alkalizing. Eat to your health!

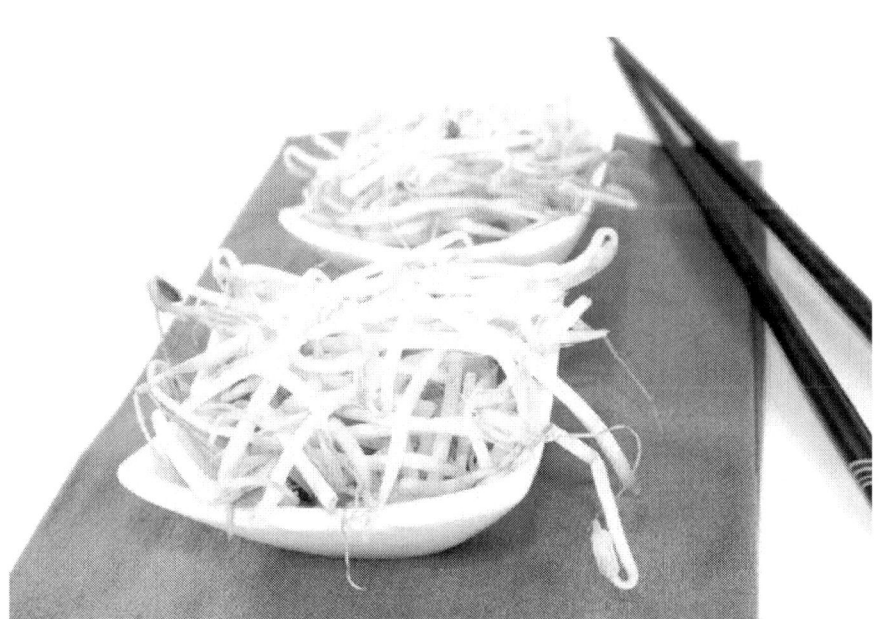

Raw Veggie Noodles

I really recommend that you get a spiralizer. It's amazing how much it can help you to create meals that are not only healthy but also visually appealing. Just have a look at this simple vegetable salad in the form of veggie noodles.

Serves: 2

Ingredients:

- 4 carrots
- 2 cucumbers
- 1 zucchini
- 1 tablespoon of coconut oil
- A few cilantro leaves
- ½ cup radish
- ¼ cup of dried fruit of your choice
- 1 avocado, peeled, pitted and sliced
- Organic, cold-pressed virgin olive oil
- Apple cider vinegar or lemon juice
- Himalaya salt

Instructions:

1. First, place carrots, cucumbers and zucchini through a spiralizer to create a noodle-like shape.

2. Place carrots, cucumbers, dried fruits and avocado in a salad bowl.
3. Now, stir-fry the zucchini noodles in coconut oil using extremely low heat. You just want zucchini to soften up a bit and absorb the coconut flavor.
4. When done, add zucchini into the salad bowl and mix well with other ingredients.
5. Sprinkle some olive oil, lemon juice or vinegar over the salad.
6. Season with Himalayan salt and garnish with cilantro leaves.
7. Enjoy!

Coconut Gazpacho-Style Raw Veggie Cream

This is an oriental, spiced-up version of traditional Spanish gazpacho. I like to add some wakame seaweed because it's extremely nutritious. It is rich in Vitamin A, Vitamin C, Vitamin E, Vitamin K, Niacin, Pantothenic Acid, Phosphorus, Calcium, Iron, Magnesium, and Manganese.

Of course, it's not a must-have ingredient to enjoy this recipe. It's totally optional, but if you haven't tried wakame, I really encourage you to put it on your shopping list. It is certainly one of my favorite super foods, and it's not that expensive, because you only use a few inches of it at a time!

Serves: 2

Ingredients:

- 4 big tomatoes, peeled (immersing them in warm water will help remove peel)
- 2 big cucumbers
- 2 garlic cloves
- 1 cup coconut milk
- 2 tablespoons of coconut oil (slightly melted)
- ¼ cup cilantro
- ½ teaspoon turmeric
- ¼ teaspoon black pepper

- A few mint leaves
- 1 square inches of wakame seaweed, soaked in water
- Himalayan salt to taste

Instructions:

1. Place all the ingredients (aside from salt, spices, and coconut oil) in a blender.
2. After blending, mix in some coconut oil, Himalayan salt, and spices. Stir well.
3. Enjoy!

Almost Raw Curry

The raw food diet is not only about totally raw foods. It's OK to either steam your foods slightly or do a bit of stir-frying on low heat. You already know the rule- just don't exceed 100° Fahrenheit.

Aside from that, you can add this recipe to some cooked food to make it healthier. Here's my tip to help you save some time- cook some quinoa or basmati rice in batches and freeze them. Then, if you want a healthy, delicious meal, it will only take a few minutes to prepare an almost raw veggie curry that you can serve with pretty much everything: other raw food meals, rice, or quinoa. If you follow something like a Paleo Diet, you could add it to your fish or meat. It all depends on your personal choices and nutritional lifestyle preferences. In this book, I want to accommodate all of you- vegans, alkalarians, vegetarians, Paleos, and those who follow their own diet- by mixing different philosophies together.

Serves: 2

Ingredients:

- 2 carrots, sliced thinly (I suggest you use a spiralizer for perfectly thin slices)

- 2 zucchini, also cut into small slices (place through a spiralizer)
- 1 onion, sliced in rings
- 1 cup spinach leaves
- Coconut oil
- Coconut milk
- Curry powder
- Ginger powder
- Himalayan salt

Instructions:

1. Start by stir-frying onion rings in coconut oil (medium heat).
2. When turning golden, reduce the heat to low heat.
3. Now add the spinach, carrots and zucchini.
4. Add spices, coconut milk, and salt.
5. Keep stir frying on low heat. You just want it to get a bit softer so don't overdo.
6. Turn off the heat, place on a plate, and sprinkle some cilantro and fresh lime juice over the curry.
7. Enjoy!

Alkaline Raw Green Energy Juice

Really simple and refreshing! I strongly recommend this recipe to those of you who are new to juicing vegetables and need to get used to the way they taste. In order to make the transition, I always recommend adding some apples and carrots. Usually, I am not a big fan of fruit juices. I only use fruits in smoothies, or I just eat them. However, you can add them to your vegetable juices for a better taste. This recipe is a perfect example!

Ginger will give your juices a nice, oriental taste. Don't forget about its benefits: it helps balance your pH, acts as a natural anti-inflammatory, and helps strengthen your immune system.

Serves: 2

Ingredients:

- 2 big cucumbers, peeled and sliced
- 1 big green apple
- 4 carrots, peeled
- A few inches of ginger
- 1 cup of spinach or kale (make sure you wash well in clean, filtered water)
- 1 teaspoon maca powder

Instructions:

1. Extract juices using a low speed juicer.
2. Stir in some maca powder and enjoy the natural energy boost!

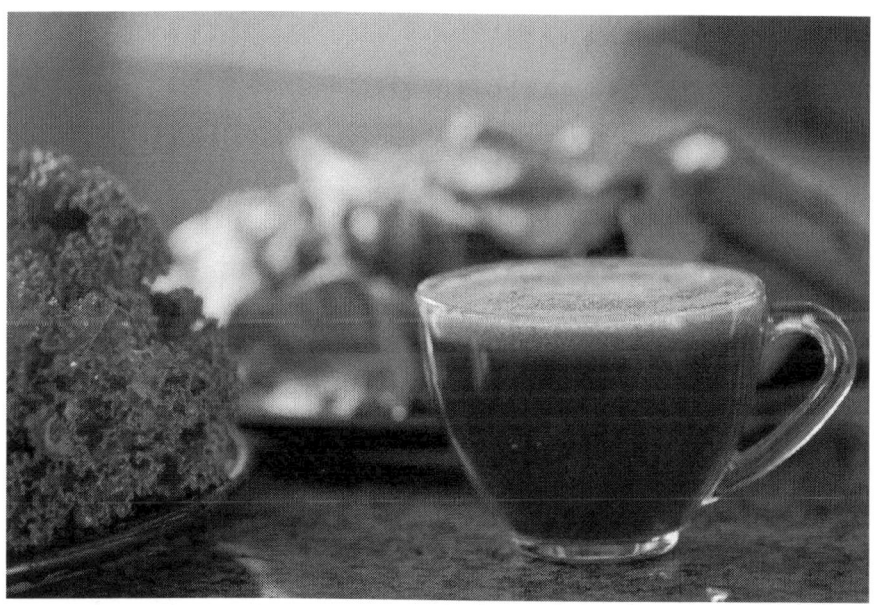

Liver Lover Green-ish Juice

Juicing vegetables is an amazing way to give your mind and body a natural energy boost! You don't need to rely on caffeine. You can actually feed your body with natural, chlorophyll rich vegetable juices, so that you achieve real energy with no side effects that usually accompany excessive caffeine consumption (headaches, migraines, acidity, insomnia, irritability, PMS). Get committed to drinking one raw vegetable juice a day, and you will be amazed by the results!

In order to define the taste and make your vegetable juices more appealing, experiment with spices and herbs. The easiest way is to add some Himalayan salt. By the way, Himalayan salt is nothing you should fear; it's good for you. Simple lesson learned- there are good salts and bad salts just like there are good fats and bad fats. Himalayan salt has multiple health and wellness benefits, including:

- It helps strengthen the bones (it has some mineral content like: magnesium, calcium, potassium)
- Improves circulation
- Prevents muscle cramps
- Balances pH, helping prevent acid reflux
- Helps create an electrolyte balance

Serves: 1

Ingredients:

- 3 cups of romaine lettuce, cleansed in filtered water
- 1 bell pepper
- 2 big tomatoes
- 1 zucchini
- 1 garlic clove
- A few radishes
- Olive Oil (virgin, organic, cold-pressed)
- Himalayan Salt

Instructions:

1. Extract the juice using a low speed juicer (like Omega juicer that I am using).
2. Mix in 1 tablespoon of olive oil for better absorption. You can also use some other oil like avocado, coconut, flaxseed, etc.
3. Add some Himalayan salt for better taste.
4. Enjoy!

Refreshing Mango Blend

Why do I love coconut water, and why should you love it as well?

It's simple; coconut water stands out as a natural, alkaline drink that:

-provides optimal hydration

-is rich in potassium

-is low in calories (as you already know I am not that obsessed about calories, but I guess this is a good benefit for some of you to know)

-helps improve digestion

-is a great natural remedy for hangovers (good thing to know, right?)

-is packed with calcium, magnesium, phosphorous, potassium and sodium.

Now, let's turn theory into practice!

Serves: 2

Ingredients:

- 2 cups of watermelon (diced)
- 1 cup of mango (diced)
- 1 tablespoon alfalfa powder
- 1 cup of coconut water
- 1 teaspoon of powdered ginger
- ¼ cup of parsley leaves

Instructions:

Blend and enjoy!

Delicious Choco-Vegan Shake

Serves: 1-2

Ingredients:

- 2 bananas
- A few pineapple slices
- 2 tablespoons raw cacao
- 1 tablespoon coconut oil
- 1 cup raw almond milk
- Some raw vanilla powder to taste (optional)

Instructions:

Blend and enjoy!

Body and Mind Energizing Roibos Berry Treat

This creamy mix is a great, healthy dessert or snack option. Roibos tea is a rather unusual smoothie ingredient, but trust me; it blends well! Try it yourself.

Besides, it's a great source of Magnesium and Iron. I also like using it as a coffee or black tea substitute. Ever since I switched to a more natural diet and lifestyle, and I added more raw foods into my diet, I realized I did not need to resort to caffeine for energy!

Serves: 2

Ingredients:

- 1 cup roibos tea, cooled down
- ½ cup almond milk
- ½ cup strawberries
- ½ cup blueberries
- Juice of 2 lemons
- ¼ cup of raisins

Instructions:

Blend and enjoy!

Raw Vegan Green-ish Yoghurt

This creamy smoothie tastes a bit like Greek Yoghurt. The good news is that it's vegan friendly, dairy free, raw, natural, and unfermented.

Serves: 2

Ingredients:

- 1 banana
- 1 avocado
- 1 glass raw almond milk
- Juice of 1 lemon
- 2 tablespoons of coconut oil

Instructions:

Blend well and enjoy!

Sweet Choco-Avo Pudding

Serves: 2

Ingredients:

- 1 big avocado
- 2 tablespoons of raw cacao powder
- ¼ cup almonds (soaked)
- 1 teaspoon maca powder
- 1 teaspoon ginger powder
- Stevia to sweeten (optional)

Instructions:

1. Blend well and enjoy!
2. I really like to serve this recipe with some fresh fruit salads, especially berries and strawberries. Such a mix gives me an incredible boost of energy; try it!

Raw Orange Ice-Cream

What's the point of buying some artificial, diary ice cream that is packed with chemicals (and what's worse- uses animal products) if you can make your own that is packed with vitamins and minerals?

Serves: 2

Ingredients:

- 3 oranges, peeled
- 1/2 cup Macadamia nuts (soaked in water for a few hours)
- ½ cup coconut milk
- Cinnamon and stevia to taste
- 2 tablespoons coconut oil

Instructions:

1. Blend all the ingredients, add some coconut oil, and stir well.
2. Scoop into ice cream dishes and place in a freezer.
3. Wait a few hours and enjoy!

Vegan Raw Brownies

If you want to satisfy your sweet tooth, you have come to the right place. There are many healthy options out there, and they are much more nutritious than mainstream processed and packaged sweets.

You see, if you want to go healthy, you don't have to go hungry or survive on broccoli and kale. Simply choose natural, unprocessed ingredients. This recipe will show you what I do!

Serves: 2

Ingredients:

- 1 cup walnuts (soaked in water)
- 1 cup raw cacao powder
- A few fresh mint leaves
- ½ cup dried dates (pitted)
- 2 tablespoons coconut milk or cream
- 2 tablespoons coconut oil

Instructions:

1. Blend in a food processor or a blender.
2. Make sure the consistency is thick.

3. Form brownies and place them in a container.
4. Put in a fridge for a few hours.
5. Garnish with some mint leaves.
6. Serve and enjoy!

Amazing Alkaline Ginger Cookies

Many people associate the raw food diet with heaps of salads, but who said you cannot enjoy some natural treats? These cookies are vegan and gluten-free. Unlike modern, processed sweets that are packed with tons of chemicals and other artificial ingredients we should avoid, the treat I am about to teach you is all natural. Besides, spices and herbs have anti-inflammatory and alkalizing properties.

Almonds are definitely my favorite nut. If you have downloaded my free guide on the Alkaline Diet (it also includes alkaline-acid charts), you will see that almonds have alkalizing properties. Some people worry too much about calories. For example, they make the mistake of choosing some low calorie artificial soda drink over natural, raw almond milk. However, they forget that what really matters are nutrients. We don't want to poison our bodies with processed crap and chemicals. This is something that our bodies were not designed to eat (I am thinking Paleo here!). Anyway, let's discuss almonds and almond milk in the next recipe. For now, enjoy your treats.

As for the guide I mentioned earlier, you can get it here:

www.holisticwellnessproject.com/alkaline

Ingredients:

Serves: 2-3

- 2 cups of powdered almonds
- 1 cup pitted dates
- ½ cup raisins
- ½ teaspoon vanilla powder (natural, organic)
- 2 tablespoons maple syrup
- 2 tablespoons coconut oil (liquefied)
- 1 tablespoon raw cocoa powder
- Optional- 1 tablespoon maca powder

Instructions:

1. Place all the ingredients in a high speed blender. Blend well.
2. Form mini cookies.
3. Place in a food container of your choice, cover it, and place in a fridge.
4. Cookies will be ready to eat after a few hours.
5. This is a great summer treat, and kids really love it (I don't have my own, but I been experimenting with my friends').

Raw Almond Milk

Of all vegan milk we can create, almond milk is certainly my favorite. Personally, I am not a big fan of soy milk, because large amounts don't agree with my stomach (even though I have always stuck to organic options). I have also experimented with rice milk, but I finally discovered an even more natural, nutritious, and raw (aside from coconut milk that I always praise) is raw almond milk. You can make your own and save money. Besides, if you make your own, you always know its ingredients. I remember looking for almond milk in bio supermarkets and in organic stores where I live. To my disappointment, most of them had added sugar (even though they had an "organic" label on them), and those that didn't were extremely expensive. This predicament has driven me to create my own rituals and make my own almond milk. Try it yourself! Almond milk is also Paleo-friendly (for those of you who follow Paleo) while soy milk and rice milk aren't. Still, when I was starting on my dairy-free journey, I would try different options to see what worked for me. Lesson learned-almond milk rocks!

After you have created this recipe, store your milk in a fridge. Almond milk will keep up to one week.

Serves: 4 cups

Ingredients:

- 4 cups filtered, preferably alkaline water
- 1 cup of raw almonds
- ½ teaspoon Himalayan salt or sea salt
- A few dates or 2 tablespoons of maple syrup

Instructions:

1. First, soak almonds in water with ½ salt (sea salt or Himalayan salt) for about 12 hours.
2. Place in a high speed blender until the mixture is smooth.
3. Strain using cheesecloth.
4. Place in a blender again, adding some pitted dates or maple syrup.
5. Stir well and place in a fridge.
6. Serve with a splash of lemon or lime juice or some fresh cinnamon. So yummy, healthy and nutritious!

Raw Coconut Milk

I realize that some people may be allergic to nuts, or for whatever reason, don't like them. I want to invite you to try some homemade raw coconut milk instead. Just like almond milk, you can use it in cooking, baking, smoothies, and other natural drinks. You can experiment with cocoa, vanilla, dried fruits, and strawberries to give it some flavor.

Serves: 4

Ingredients:

- 4 cups of warm water
- 2 cups shredded coconut

Instructions:

1. I recommend you make this recipe in 2 batches.
2. First, take 1 cup of coconut and 2 cups of water and place in a blender. Keep blending for a few minutes until smooth.
3. Strain using a colander and set aside. Keep the strained coconut as well. You can use it for desserts or add it back to your milk.

4. Now, blend the second batch. Place another 2 cups of water and 1 cup of shredded coconut in the blender.
5. Blend well.
6. Mix the two batches and, if needed, add some of the blended coconut for more thickness.
7. Sweeten with stevia, maple syrup or blend again with some dried fruit.
8. Enjoy!

Raw Carrot Cookies

Carrots are healthy and cheap. It's amazing how many raw meals can be prepared with them. This recipe is a raw alternative to a traditional carrot cake. Feel free to experiment with different spices and flavors. Since there is no baking included, this recipe is stress-free and is not time-consuming! Whenever juicing carrots, don't throw away the pulp. You can use it later.

Serves: 4

Ingredients:

- 2 carrots, peeled and chopped finely
- Pulp from 6 carrots (juice 6 carrots before making this recipe and drink the juice to give your body some energy to proceed)
- 1 cup of oats
- 1 cup dates, pitted
- ½ cup almond powder or coconut powder
- Cinnamon, nutmeg. and cane sugar to sweeten
- 2 tablespoons coconut oil (liquefied)
- 1 cup of filtered water

Instructions:

1. Blend all the ingredients in a high speed blender or food processor.
2. Add more water if needed but remember to keep it thick.
3. Form little cookies and place in a fridge for a few hours.
4. Enjoy!

Apple and Celery Root Salad

Serves: 2-3

Ingredients:

- 1 medium red apple, diced
- 2 tablespoons of *raw mayonnaise (check the recipe below)*
- 1 medium sized celery root, peeled and grated
- 4 tablespoons of chopped walnuts
- Juice of 1 lemon
- 2 fresh scallions, sliced
- 2 tablespoons of coconut cream
- 1/4th cup of minced fresh parsley leaves

Instructions:

1. Toss celery root with diced apples and lemon juice.
2. Add the scallions, walnuts, and parsley. Toss again to combine.
3. Mix the mayonnaise with coconut yoghurt in another bowl.
4. Add the mayonnaise salad dressing to the apple mixture and toss to combine.
5. Store in a fridge for a couple of hours. Serve chilled.

*How to make Vegan Mayo

Mix: half cup almond or coconut milk, 2 tablespoons fresh lemon juice, 1 tablespoon vegan mustard, half cup of olive oil, pinch of salt and pepper. You can experiment with the consistency by adding some almond powder and coconut oil. Enjoy!

Summer Veggies Party

Serves: 4
Ingredients:

- 1 red organic beetroot, peeled and sliced
- 6 whole radishes, sliced
- 1 beetroot, peeled and sliced
- 1/2 of a red onion, peeled and sliced
- 2 small zucchini, sliced and steamed to soften up
- 1 small kohlrabi, sliced
- 1 red pepper, deseeded and sliced
- ¼ cup of sunflower seeds

Dressing:
- 2 tablespoons of olive oil (extra virgin)
- 2 teaspoons of fresh oregano, chopped
- 1 clove of garlic, peeled and finely chopped
- 1 teaspoon of organic maple syrup
- 1 tablespoon of fresh parsley leaves, chopped
- Fresh juice of 1 lemon
- Himalayan salt to taste

Instructions:
1. To make the dressing, whisk some olive oil with 1 clove of chopped garlic and maple syrup.
2. Add lemon juice, sea salt, parsley, and oregano.
3. Whisk again to combine.
4. Set aside in a fridge while you are preparing the salad.
5. Mix the sliced veggies in a big bowl.
6. Add some sunflower seeds and drizzle the salad dressing on top to serve the salad.

Green Papaya Salad Spiced Up

Papaya is just like avocado; its taste is soft and neutral. You can combine it with spice, salty, or sweet flavors. It's great for digestion, and its nutritional benefits speak for itself: papaya is a fantastic source of potassium, Vitamin A, Vitamin C and Folate. Adding more papaya into your diet will help ease digestion (it's great for irritable bowel syndrome), strengthen your immune system, and detoxify your body.

Servings: 3-4

Ingredients:
- 1 cup mixed fresh lettuce leaves
- 1 small green papaya, julienned
- ½ cup whole radish, sliced
- 2 carrots, peeled and spiralized (or sliced thinly)
- 1/ 2 cup of raw cashew nuts
- 1 cup cherry tomatoes, halved

For the Chili Spicy Dressing:
- 1 tablespoon of raw coconut vinegar
- 1 tablespoon of cane sugar or maple syrup
- 1 red long chili, seeded and finely chopped
- Juice of 2 limes
- 1 small clove of garlic, peeled and minced

Instructions:

1. Whisk all the dressing ingredients in a small bowl. Set aside in a fridge to cool.
2. In the meantime, prepare the salad by tossing all the salad ingredients together in a salad bowl.
3. Now mix the salad with the dressing so that all ingredients are equally covered.
4. Serve with some lemon wedges. Enjoy!

Rainbow Raw Salad

How can one get bored with salads if there is always so much to explore?

Serves: 3

Ingredients:

- 1 whole cucumber, diced without peeling
- 1 teaspoon of vegan mustard (optional)
- 3/4 cup of purple cabbage, chopped
- ½ teaspoon of onion powder
- 1 tablespoon of coconut vinegar
- 1 tablespoon olive oil
- 2 teaspoons of maple syrup
- 1 medium sized ripe tomato, diced
- 1 teaspoon of dill
- A pinch of garlic sea salt
- A pinch of ground black pepper

Instructions:

1. Chop the vegetables (cabbage, tomato and cucumber) and mix in a bowl.
2. Add the dressing (syrup, sea salt, pepper, vinegar and olive oil) and mix well.
3. Serve the salad right away. Enjoy!

Minty Zucchini Dream Universal Dip

I love all kinds of dips and hummus-style dishes. Of course, since this is a raw food-ish book, don't expect cooked goods or legumes. Let's turn to veggies and 100% raw options. Again, you don't have to eat raw all the time. Your goal should be to discover new raw options and try to add them into your daily diet in an enjoyable and virtually effort-free way. Taste is the mother of invention!

This dip works well as a snack with some raw veggies as well as a cold or lightly warm, creamy soup. You can also use it in wraps, on rice dishes, and in curry dishes.

Serves: 2

Ingredients:

- 2 zucchini, peeled
- ¼ cup fresh mint leaves
- ¼ cup fresh cilantro leaves
- 1 teaspoon turmeric powder
- ½ teaspoon black pepper powder
- ½ teaspoon cilantro powder
- 1/2 cup coconut milk
- 1 lime

- Himalayan salt to taste

Instructions:

1. Blend in a high speed blender or a food processor in order to obtain a smooth, creamy consistency.
2. Squeeze in some lime juice and add Himalayan salt to taste.
3. Enjoy!

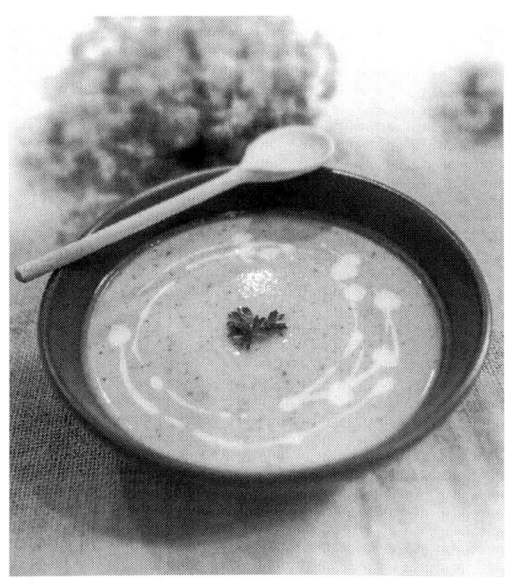

Papaya Guacamole Spiced Up

Papaya is a great alternative to avocado, and I really recommend that you eat more of this interesting fruit, especially if you want to ease your digestive problems. This recipe will give you an idea of how to create, not only a deliciously tasting and healthy snack, but also a visually appealing orange guacamole-style dip. Dips are some of my raw food staples. They are easy to make, and they make my blender work really, really hard (it actually enjoys working overtime).

Serves: 2

Ingredients:

- 1 small papaya fruit
- 2 big tomatoes, peeled (put in some warm water so as to peel easily)
- 2 tablespoon olive oil
- Juice of 2 limes
- Himalayan Salt
- Pinch of curry powder and black pepper

Instructions:

1. Blend and enjoy!

2. Serve with some raw or slightly steamed veggies.
3. You can also add some nuts and seeds.

Healthy Eyes Raw Juice

I must admit that when I first heard about juicing sweet potatoes, I thought it was something more than weird. I remember that one of my massage therapy teachers, who also happened to be a naturopathy teacher, was telling me all about it. Even though I still thought it was rather unusual (at that time I was making the mistake of drinking processed, sugary fruit juices), I decided to leave my comfort zone and try it. So should you. In case you are not new to juicing sweet potatoes, I hope that relaying the health benefits of these practices will be your motivator to continue. These include:

- Eye care (the sweet potato juice is rich in Vitamin A)
- Natural anti-age (it is full of Vitamin E)
- Can help prevent cancer and Alzheimer's disease (it is rich in quercetin and, according to the journal "Cancer Science," quercetin stops the progression of tumors associated with skin cancer)

Serves: 1-2

Ingredients:

- 2 sweet potatoes
- 3 carrots (peel if not organic)
- 1 green apple to taste
- 1 zucchini

- 1 tablespoon of olive oil
- Juice of ½ lemon

Instructions:

1. Juice all the ingredients using a low-speed juicer.
2. Add some lemon juice and olive oil (it will help your body absorb the nutrients from the juice) and enjoy!

I often get asked what to do with the pulp; very few people want to throw it away. I recommend that you add it to your soups or salads, or you can use it for baking or making pancakes. You can also add it to vegetable curries. Personally, I don't like throwing away the pulp of highly nutritious, and very often a bit expensive, fruits and vegetables. More on that later!

Drink It Up- Health Shot!

To be honest, I am not a great broccoli lover (this is something I discuss in my course, AlkalineDietLifestyle.com), however, I discovered that juicing it is a different story. The way I see it, toughen up and get your health shot!

Who would have thought of a Polish girl drinking broccoli juice shots?

Why do I do it? It's simple; I want to invest in my health, and I know that one green juice a day will keep a doctor away! This is a fantastic, natural anti-age, and vibrant health recipe, and it also helps cleanse the liver (liver lovers club).

Serves: 1-2

Ingredients:

- 1 broccoli, chopped
- A few inches of ginger
- Juice of 1 lemon
- 1 tablespoon olive oil

Instructions:

1. Extract the juices using a low speed juicer.
2. Add some lemon juice and olive oil, and drink it up!

MY TIP

Now, why would I throw away the pulp of my super healthy, organic broccoli? It's full of nutrients and natural fiber. It's great for gluten-free recipes. I suggest you keep the pulp and add it to your soups and salads.

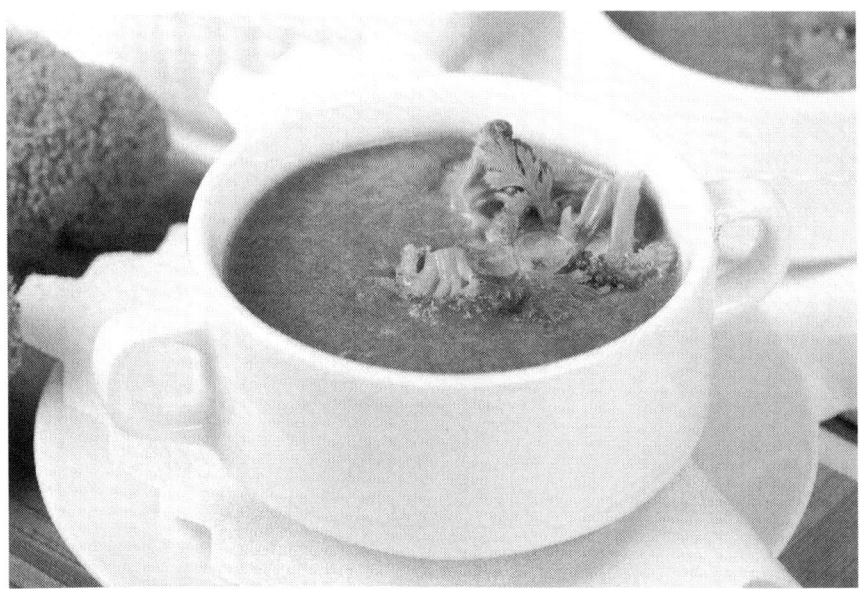

Sweet Juice

Trying to fight sugar cravings in a natural way? Try this recipe. To be honest, I am not a big fan of beets, however, juiced beets are a different story!

Serves: 1-2

Ingredients:

- 2 beetroots (peel, unless they are organic)
- 2 carrots (no need to peel if organic)
- Juice of 1/2 lemon
- 1 tablespoon olive oil or avocado oil

Instructions:

1. Extract juices using a low-speed juicer.
2. Add some lemon juice and olive oil and enjoy!
3. If you don't want to add oils, you can also add some avocado or simply snack on some nuts. As I always try to remind you, if you accompany your juice with some healthy nuts, it's a real game changer. Try it!

Extra tips:

Since beets are full of polysaccharide-rich fiber, I recommend you keep the pulp and use it for soups, creams, salsas and salads. It's also great for baking.

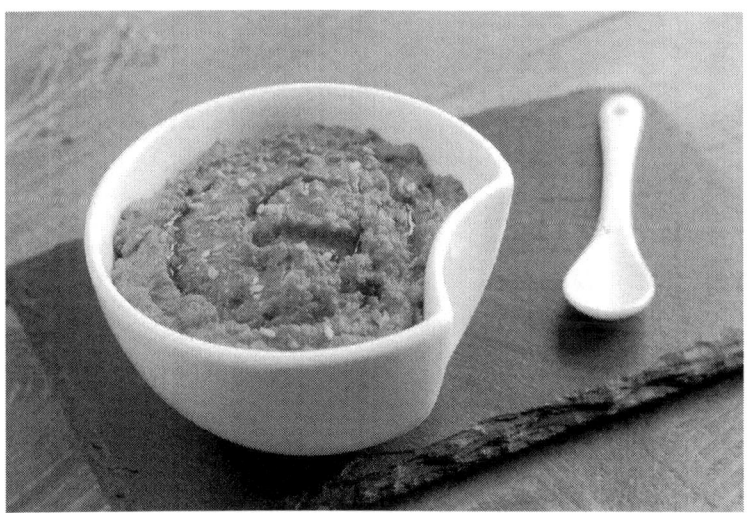

Holiday Feeling Tropical Anti-Inflammatory Juice

Are you looking for some refreshment and relaxation? Try this recipe. It smells and tastes fantastic! Its rich bromelain content will help with digestive problems, cellulite battles, and inflammation.

Serves: 1-2

Ingredients:

- 8 slices of pineapple
- 2 carrots
- A few inches of ginger
- 1 orange
- ½ cup water

Instructions:

1. Extract juices from all the ingredients.
2. Add water, stir well, add some ice cubes, and serve.
3. Enjoy and snack on a few nuts to stimulate better nutrient absorption.

OK, I can hear some questions and voices of confusion here...

"But, Marta, juicing is expensive! I need to buy lots of fruits to only get a couple of glasses of juice. What do I do with the pulp?"

I totally agree, and I was thinking the same. What's the point of wasting your food, especially good quality, wholesome food? This is why I decided to experiment. The following bonus recipe is one of the results I have gotten so far (my recipe beta testers enjoyed it, and it's 100% raw!). You can also use it as a template for other kinds of pulp.

Ingredients:

- Pulp from our pineapple anti-inflammatory juice
- 2 scallions (green onions)
- ¼ cup of cilantro, finely chopped
- 0.5 inch chili pepper, or a pinch of chili pepper powder (add more if you want it super spicy)
- 2 tablespoons of coconut milk
- Juice of 1 lime
- Pinch of curry powder
- 1 tablespoon avocado oil or olive oil

Instructions:

1. Blend in a high-speed blender or a food processor until smooth.
2. Serve with raw veggies, rice, and in wraps.
3. Enjoy! It's tasty and healthy.

Longevity Sweet Juice 2 in 1 Recipe

This recipe will show you how to create vegetable juices with an amazing taste and use the pulp. This is like a 2 in 1 raw vegan treat recipe!

Serves: 2-3

Ingredients:

- 2 beetroots, peeled unless organic
- 2 red bell peppers
- 2 carrots, peeled unless organic
- 1 cucumber, peeled
- 2 inches of ginger, peeled
- ½ red cabbage

Instructions:

1. Extract juices in a low speed juicer.
2. Add some healthy oil or snack on a few nuts for better absorption. Another option is to add an avocado. The choice is yours.

BONUS Recipe- What to do with a pulp?

Create some sweet, grain free, gluten free, raw, dairy free, and vegan friendly treats that you can spread on your fruits (tastes great of apple slices), or quinoa. You can also use it as a quick snack. If you store it in a fridge, it will keep up to 3 days. It actually gets better after a day or two.

Serves: 2-3

Ingredients:

- Pulp from the previous recipe
- 3 tablespoons of maple syrup
- 2 tablespoons coconut milk
- 1 teaspoon cinnamon powder
- 1 teaspoon ginger powder
- 1 cup pitted dates
- 2 tablespoons coconut oil

Instructions:

1. Blend until smooth and place in a jar.
2. Put in a fridge and serve cold.
3. Enjoy!

Additional tips:

You can also use the pulp to create a spicy recipe. Simply blend some onions, cilantro, olive oil, and spices into to pulp. Enjoy!

Mango Mustard Salad

If you invest time in creating a myriad of mouth-watering salad dressings, you will never get bored with raw food salads! My tip is to always make salsas and salads in batches. You can store them in your fridge so that you always have some delicious and nutritious raw foods to grab. This simple strategy will save you time and money, and you will be able to avoid temptations like eating out or choosing unhealthy options. Healthy and stress-free solutions on a budget!

Serves: 2

Ingredients (Salad):

- 2 cups iceberg lettuce, chopped
- 1 cup cherry tomato, cut in halves
- 1 big cucumber, sliced and peeled
- 2 tablespoon chai seeds
- 1 garlic clove

Ingredients (Salsa):

- 2 teaspoons tahini
- ½ cup mango, chopped
- 2 teaspoons raw, vegan mustard
- 1 tablespoon raw apple cider vinegar

- ½ cup cashews, powdered
- Himalayan salt to taste

Instructions:

1. First, blend all the salad dressing ingredients. Stir well.
2. Put in a fridge and get started on your salad.
3. Place all the salad ingredients in a salad bowl and mix well.
4. Add the salsa and season with Himalayan salt.
5. Enjoy!

More Delicious Salad Dressings and Salsas

Raw Italian Salad Dressing

Mix:
- 2 tablespoons olive oil
- Juice of 1 lemon
- 2 tablespoons of apple cider vinegar
- ¼ cup flax oil
- 1 teaspoon oregano
- ¼ onion
- 1 teaspoon basil
- Himalayan salt to taste
- ½ teaspoon garlic powder

Alkaline Thyme Salad Dressing

Mix:
- Juice of 1 lemon
- 2 tablespoons of olive oil
- 1 teaspoon dried basil
- 1 tablespoon fresh thyme
- 1 teaspoon alfalfa powder
- Himalayan salt to taste

Creamy Spinach Salad Dressing

Blend:
- 1 cup spinach
- 2 garlic cloves
- Juice of 1 lemon
- ½ cup coconut milk
- ¼ cup cashews
- ¼ teaspoon nutmeg
- Himalayan salt and black pepper to taste

CONCLUSION

I hope that you enjoyed reading my recipes and have already chosen a few of them to try sometime soon. People who make at least 60-70% of their diet raw benefit from:

- Weight loss
- Brighter skin and healthier hair
- More energy levels
- More zest for life
- Less infections and colds
- Focused mind

If you decide to do raw foods part-time (by saying part-time, I mean that you will be eating 50-70% raw), remember to make the remaining non-raw, or "cooked" part as healthy as possible, and eliminate all the processed foods. I think that as soon as you try eating raw at least part-time, and you go for natural, organic foods, you will start experiencing some really amazing health benefits that will make you hooked on a healthy lifestyle.

If you are new to raw foods, I suggest you invest some money in the following utensils and equipment; they will make your life easier and save your time:

- High speed blender
- Hand Blender (excellent when you travel)
- Juicer (low speed is better as it preserves nutrients)
- Spiral Slicer
- Food Processor
- Sprouter

The question I very often get asked is:

What is better/healthier- juices or smoothies?

Here's my tip (especially for weight loss and getting rid of sugar cravings)- avoid fruit juices, with the exception of non-sugary fruits like lemons, limes, grapefruits, and tomatoes. Most juices are pure sugar and no fiber. Focus on vegetable juices, instead. You can add a bit of fruits to your vegetable juices to taste and help make the transition (this is what my recipes teach you).

Juicing is recommended to those who have a sensitive digestive system or illness that inhibits your body from processing fiber. Since there is no fiber, you only get nutrients, and your body does not need extra energy to digest it. This is why juicing vegetables first thing in the morning is so beneficial for your health, in addition to giving you a real energy boost.

Why you should avoid fruit juices (even home-made):

We already know that most fruits contain sugar, so imagine what happens when you juice them... When you remove the fiber, the liquid juice is absorbed into your blood stream much quicker than it does with fiber. This is why, if you are juicing fruits, it will lead to unstable blood sugar levels and a drop in blood sugar. This can cause low energy levels and sugar cravings. Drinking pure fruit juices will make you hungry, and your body will ask for sugar to add to the vicious cycle...

Exception: You can have an occasional orange juice, but make sure you dilute it in some water. Pure orange juice is not that good for you, especially if you want to lose weight.

Smoothies are a different story, because when you blend fruit, you also get fiber. So when you drink it, your body says 'no' when you are full. Fruit smoothies are natural, raw and nutritious.

To sum up - juicing - yes, but juice vegetables and non-sugary fruit.

Blending - yes, it's also good for you and smoothies will make you feel full longer. However, if you can't tolerate too much fiber because of any specific digestive problems, go for juicing first.

For more wellness inspiration and empowerment visit the blog:

www.holisticwellnessproject.com

Don't forget to grab your 3 free eBooks:

www.HolisticWellnessProject.com/alkaline

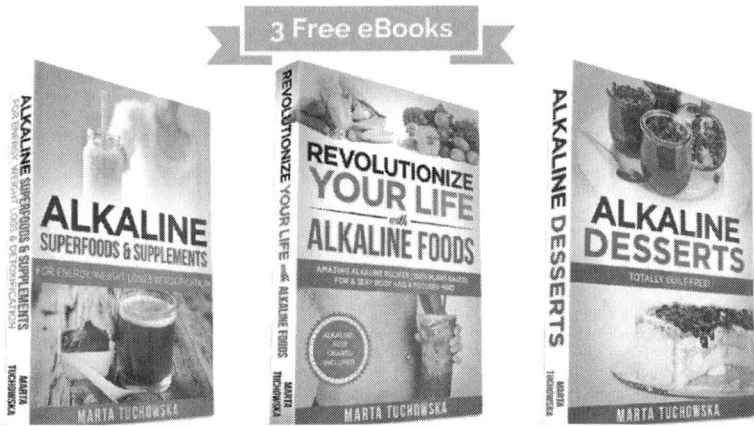

If you have any questions, doubts, or you find my instructions confusing and need more guidance, please e-mail me at:

Info@holisticwellnessproject.com

I receive tons of e-mails from my readers every day, and I am always more than happy to help them. It's you I am writing for and I would love to hear from you.

To check out more of my books on Amazon, please visit:

www.holisticwellnessproject.com/books

PLEASE POST A REVIEW

Finally, if you enjoyed my book and you feel like it has helped you and inspired you towards a healthier nutrition, please let others know! Simply post your review on Amazon.

Thanks in advance for your time and interest in my work.

It was a pleasure to "talk" to you,

I hope we "meet" again soon!

I wish you wellness, health, and success in whatever it is that you want to accomplish.

Marta

Connect with me:

www.facebook.com/HolisticWellnessProject

www.twitter.com/Marta_Wellness

www.pinterest.com/martaWellness/

Made in the USA
Columbia, SC
17 November 2018